MENTAL HEALTH DIET COOKBOOK

Mary Dixon

TABLE OF CONTENT

CHAPTER ONE

Mental Health Diet and Benefits

Following a mental health diet can have significant benefits for your overall well-being. Here's a step-by-step guide on how to do it:

1. Consult a Healthcare Professional: Before making any significant changes to your diet, consult a healthcare professional, such as a doctor or a registered dietitian. They can assess your specific needs and provide personalized recommendations.

2. Embrace Whole, Nutrient-Dense Foods:

- Fruits and Vegetables: Incorporate a variety of colorful fruits and vegetables into your daily meals. They are rich in vitamins, minerals, and antioxidants that support mental health.

- Whole Grains: Choose whole grains like brown rice, quinoa, and whole wheat over refined grains. They provide steady energy and may improve mood.

- Lean Proteins: Include lean sources of protein such as poultry, fish, beans, and tofu. Protein supports the production of neurotransmitters that affect mood.

- Healthy Fats: Opt for sources of healthy fats like avocados, nuts, seeds, and fatty fish (salmon, mackerel, sardines). Omega-3 fatty acids, in particular, have been linked to improved mood and reduced anxiety.

3. Limit Processed Foods and Sugar:

- Minimize your intake of processed foods, sugary snacks, and sugary drinks. These can lead to mood swings and energy crashes.
- Reduce or eliminate artificial additives and preservatives from your diet.

4. Mindful Eating: Practice mindful eating to develop a healthier relationship with food.

- Pay attention to hunger and fullness cues.
- Savor each bite and eat slowly.
- Avoid distractions like TV or smartphones while eating.

5. Stay Hydrated: Proper hydration is crucial for mental health. Drink plenty of water throughout the day to help maintain cognitive function and mood stability.

6. Balanced Meals and Sncks:

- Eat regular, balanced meals to maintain stable blood sugar levels.
- Include healthy snacks like nuts, yogurt, or fruit to prevent extreme hunger and mood swings.

7. Limit Caffeine and Alcohol: While some people can enjoy these in moderation, excessive caffeine and alcohol consumption can negatively impact mental health. Be mindful of your intake.

8. Consider Supplements: If your healthcare professional recommends it, you may consider supplements like vitamin D, omega-3 fatty acids, or B-complex vitamins to support mental health.

9. Exercise Regularly: Incorporate physical activity into your routine. Exercise releases endorphins, which can improve mood and reduce stress.

10. Sleep Well: Prioritize quality sleep. Poor sleep can exacerbate mental health issues. Create a relaxing bedtime routine and aim for 7-9 hours of sleep per night.

11. Manage Stress: Practice stress-reduction techniques such as meditation, yoga, deep breathing exercises, or mindfulness to support mental well-being.

12. Seek Professional Help: If you're struggling with mental health issues, don't hesitate to seek help from a therapist, counselor, or psychiatrist. Dietary changes can complement therapy and medication when necessary.

Remember that a mental health diet is just one part of a holistic approach to mental well-being. Combining a nutritious diet with other lifestyle factors like regular exercise, sleep, and stress management can lead to significant improvements in your mental health and overall quality of life.

CHAPTER TWO

14-Day Mental Health Diet Meal Plan

Creating a comprehensive 14-day mental health diet meal plan involves including a variety of nutrient-rich foods that support mood and overall well-being.

Please keep in mind that this meal plan is a general guideline, and individual dietary needs may vary. Consult with a healthcare professional or registered dietitian for personalized recommendations. Here's a sample meal plan:

Day 1:

- Breakfast: Greek yogurt with berries and honey, a handful of almonds.
- Lunch: Spinach and kale salad with grilled chicken, cherry tomatoes, and balsamic vinaigrette.
- Snack: Carrot sticks with hummus.
- Dinner: Baked salmon with quinoa and steamed broccoli.

Day 2:

- Breakfast: Oatmeal topped with sliced bananas, walnuts, and a drizzle of maple syrup.
- Lunch: Whole-grain wrap with turkey, avocado, spinach, and a side of mixed greens.
- Snack: Mixed berries and a small piece of dark chocolate.
- Dinner: Stir-fried tofu with broccoli, bell peppers, and brown rice.

Day 3:

- Breakfast: Scrambled eggs with sautéed spinach and a side of whole-grain toast.
- Lunch: Lentil soup with a side of mixed greens and a whole-grain roll.
- Snack: Cottage cheese with pineapple chunks.
- Dinner: Grilled shrimp with quinoa and roasted asparagus.

Day 4:

- Breakfast: Smoothie with spinach, banana, almond milk, and a scoop of protein powder.
- Lunch: Quinoa salad with chickpeas, cucumbers, tomatoes, and feta cheese.
- Snack: Sliced cucumbers with tzatziki sauce.
- Dinner: Baked chicken breast with sweet potato and steamed green beans.

Day 5:

- Breakfast: Whole-grain cereal with low-fat milk and sliced strawberries.
- Lunch: Turkey and vegetable stir-fry with brown rice.
- Snack: A small handful of mixed nuts.
- Dinner: Grilled cod with quinoa and sautéed spinach.

Day 6:

- Breakfast: Cottage cheese with pineapple and a sprinkle of chia seeds.
- Lunch: Spinach and mushroom omelet with a side of mixed greens.

- Snack: Sliced bell peppers with guacamole.
- Dinner: Baked tofu with brown rice and roasted Brussels sprouts.

Day 7:

- Breakfast: Whole-grain pancakes with fresh blueberries and a dollop of Greek yogurt.
- Lunch: Mixed bean salad with cherry tomatoes, corn, and a lime-cilantro dressing.
- Snack: Sliced apples with almond butter.
- Dinner: Grilled chicken with quinoa and steamed broccoli.

Day 8:

- Breakfast: Greek yogurt parfait with granola, sliced strawberries, and a drizzle of honey.
- Lunch: Grilled salmon salad with mixed greens, cucumber, and a lemon-dill dressing.
- Snack: Baby carrots with a small serving of hummus.
- Dinner: Lentil and vegetable curry served over brown rice.

Day 9:

- Breakfast: Whole-grain toast with avocado and poached eggs.
- Lunch: Turkey and vegetable wrap with a side of carrot sticks.
- Snack: A handful of grapes and a piece of string cheese.
- Dinner: Baked tilapia with quinoa and roasted asparagus.

Day 10:

- Breakfast: Smoothie with spinach, mango, almond milk, and a scoop of protein powder.
- Lunch: Quinoa salad with black beans, corn, bell peppers, and a lime vinaigrette.
- Snack: Sliced cucumber with tzatziki sauce.
- Dinner: Grilled chicken breast with sweet potato and steamed green beans.

Day 11:

- Breakfast: Whole-grain cereal with low-fat milk and sliced bananas.
- Lunch: Vegetable stir-fry with tofu and brown rice.
- Snack: A small handful of mixed nuts.
- Dinner: Baked cod with quinoa and sautéed spinach.

Day 12:

- Breakfast: Cottage cheese with pineapple and a sprinkle of chia seeds.
- Lunch: Spinach and mushroom omelet with a side of mixed greens.
- Snack: Sliced bell peppers with guacamole.
- Dinner: Baked tofu with brown rice and roasted Brussels sprouts.

Day 13:

- Breakfast: Whole-grain pancakes with fresh blueberries and a dollop of Greek yogurt.
- Lunch: Mixed bean salad with cherry tomatoes, corn, and a lime-cilantro dressing.

- Snack: Sliced apples with almond butter.
- Dinner: Grilled chicken with quinoa and steamed broccoli.

Day 14:

- Breakfast: Scrambled eggs with sautéed spinach and a side of whole-grain toast.
- Lunch: Lentil soup with a side of mixed greens and a whole-grain roll.
- Snack: Cottage cheese with pineapple chunks.
- Dinner: Grilled shrimp with quinoa and roasted asparagus.

Remember that this meal plan serves as a general guideline, and you should adjust it to your individual preferences and nutritional needs. It's essential to maintain a balanced and varied diet to support your mental health effectively.

Additionally, stay hydrated, engage in regular physical activity, practice stress management, and get enough sleep to maximize the benefits of this mental health diet.

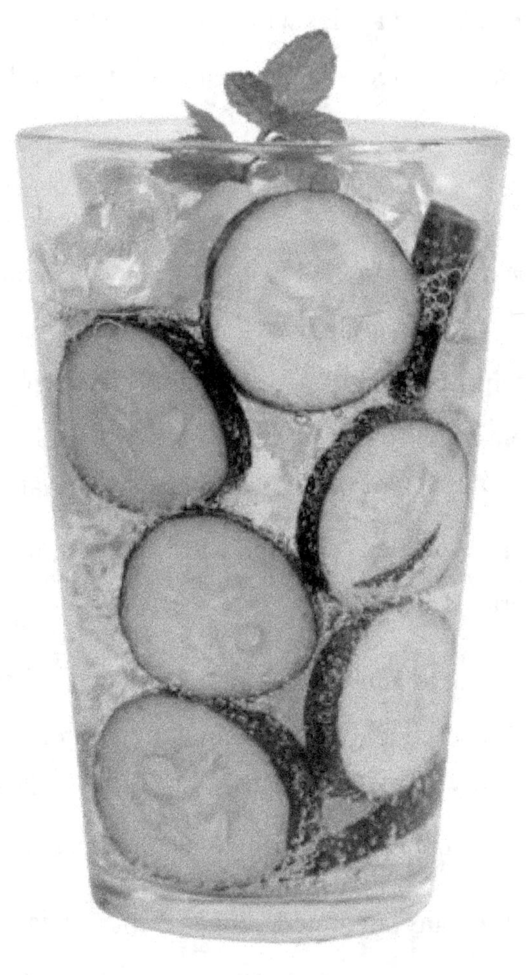

CHAPTER THREE

Mental Health Diet Breakfast Recipes

1. Berry Bliss Greek Yogurt Parfait

Start your day with a burst of antioxidants and probiotics in this delicious parfait.

Ingredients:

- 1 cup Greek yogurt
- 1/2 cup mixed berries (strawberries, blueberries, raspberries)
- 2 tablespoons honey
- 2 tablespoons granola

Instructions:

1. In a glass or bowl, layer half of the Greek yogurt.

2. Add half of the mixed berries and drizzle with honey.

3. Add the remaining yogurt and top with the rest of the berries.

4. Sprinkle granola on top.

5. Serve immediately.

Cooking Time: 5 minutes

2. Nutty Banana Oatmeal

This hearty oatmeal combines the goodness of whole grains, nuts, and bananas for a comforting breakfast.

Ingredients:

- 1/2 cup rolled oats
- 1 cup almond milk (or your choice of milk)
- 1 ripe banana, sliced
- 2 tablespoons chopped walnuts
- 1 tablespoon honey (optional)

Instructions:

1. In a saucepan, bring the almond milk to a simmer.

2. Add the oats and cook on low heat, stirring occasionally, for about 5 minutes or until the oats are tender.

3. Top with banana slices, walnuts, and a drizzle of honey, if desired.

Cooking Time: 10 minutes

3. Spinach and Mushroom Scramble

Packed with protein and nutrients, this savory scramble is a great way to incorporate greens into your morning routine.

Ingredients:

- 2 large eggs
- 1 cup fresh spinach leaves
- 1/2 cup sliced mushrooms
- Salt and pepper to taste
- 1 teaspoon olive oil

Instructions:

1. Heat olive oil in a non-stick skillet over medium heat.

2. Add mushrooms and sauté until they release moisture and turn golden brown.

3. Add spinach and cook until wilted.

4. Whisk the eggs in a bowl, season with salt and pepper, and pour into the skillet.

5. Cook, stirring gently, until the eggs are set.

Cooking Time: 10 minutes

4. Avocado Toast with Poached Egg

Creamy avocado and a perfectly poached egg make this toast a satisfying and nutritious breakfast.

Ingredients:

- 1 slice whole-grain bread
- 1/2 ripe avocado, mashed
- 1 poached egg
- Salt and pepper to taste
- Red pepper flakes (optional)

Instructions:

1. Toast the bread to your desired level of crispiness.

2. Spread the mashed avocado evenly on the toast.

3. Carefully place the poached egg on top.

4. Season with salt, pepper, and red pepper flakes, if desired.

Cooking Time: 15 minutes (including egg poaching)

5. Blueberry Banana Smoothie Bowl

This vibrant and nutritious smoothie bowl is a delightful way to start your day.

Ingredients:

- 1 frozen banana
- 1/2 cup frozen blueberries
- 1/2 cup Greek yogurt
- 1/4 cup almond milk
- Toppings: sliced bananas, fresh blueberries, chia seeds, and honey

Instructions:

1. Blend the frozen banana, frozen blueberries, Greek yogurt, and almond milk until smooth.

2. Pour the smoothie into a bowl.

3. Top with sliced bananas, fresh blueberries, chia seeds, and a drizzle of honey.

Cooking Time: 5 minutes

6. Peanut Butter and Banana Overnight Oats

Prep these oats the night before for a quick and filling breakfast that's rich in fiber and protein.

Ingredients:

- 1/2 cup rolled oats
- 1 cup almond milk (or your choice of milk)
- 2 tablespoons natural peanut butter
- 1 ripe banana, sliced
- 1 tablespoon honey

Instructions:

1. In a jar or container, combine oats and almond milk.

2. Stir in peanut butter and honey.

3. Add banana slices.

4. Cover and refrigerate overnight.

5. Give it a good stir in the morning before enjoying.

Cooking Time: 5 minutes (plus overnight chilling)

7. Veggie Breakfast Burrito

This savory breakfast burrito is filled with veggies and protein to keep you full and focused.

Ingredients:

- 2 large eggs, beaten
- 1 whole-grain tortilla
- 1/4 cup black beans, drained and rinsed
- 1/4 cup diced bell peppers
- 1/4 cup diced onions
- Salsa for topping (optional)
- Salt and pepper to taste

Instructions:

1. In a non-stick skillet, sauté the onions and bell peppers until they soften.

2. Add the beaten eggs and scramble until cooked.

3. Warm the tortilla in the skillet or microwave.

4. Lay the tortilla flat and fill with the scrambled eggs, black beans, and salsa if desired.

5. Roll up the burrito, tucking in the sides.

Cooking Time: 10 minutes

8. Chia Seed Pudding with Mixed Berries

Chia seeds are a great source of omega-3 fatty acids and fiber, making this pudding a nutritious breakfast option.

Ingredients:

- 2 tablespoons chia seeds
- 1/2 cup almond milk (or your choice of milk)
- 1/2 teaspoon vanilla extract
- 1/2 cup mixed berries (strawberries, blueberries, raspberries)

Instructions:

1. In a bowl, combine chia seeds, almond milk, and vanilla extract.

2. Stir well, cover, and refrigerate for at least 2 hours or overnight, stirring occasionally.

3. Top with mixed berries before serving.

Cooking Time: 5 minutes (plus chilling time)

9. Sweet Potato and Spinach Breakfast Hash

This hearty and colorful breakfast hash provides a variety of nutrients to support mental health.

Ingredients:

- 1 small sweet potato, peeled and diced
- 1 cup fresh spinach
- 1/4 cup diced red bell pepper
- 2 eggs
- Salt and pepper to taste
- Olive oil for cooking

Instructions:

1. Heat olive oil in a skillet over medium heat.

2. Add diced sweet potatoes and cook until they start to brown and become tender.

3. Add diced red bell pepper and continue to cook for a few minutes.

4. Stir in fresh spinach and cook until wilted.

5. Push the vegetables to one side of the skillet and crack the eggs into the other side.

6. Cook the eggs to your desired level of doneness.

7. Serve the eggs on top of the vegetable hash.

Cooking Time: 20 minutes

10. Quinoa Breakfast Bowl

Quinoa is a fantastic source of protein and complex carbohydrates, making it a great choice for a balanced breakfast.

Ingredients:

- 1/2 cup cooked quinoa
- 1/4 cup sliced almonds
- 1/4 cup diced dried apricots
- 1/2 cup plain Greek yogurt
- 1 tablespoon honey

Instructions:

1. In a bowl, layer cooked quinoa, sliced almonds, and diced dried apricots.

2. Top with Greek yogurt and drizzle with honey.

Cooking Time: 10 minutes (if quinoa is pre-cooked)

Mental Health Diet Lunch Recipes

1. Quinoa and Chickpea Salad

This vibrant salad is rich in plant-based protein and fiber, making it an excellent choice for a wholesome lunch.

Ingredients:

- 1 cup cooked quinoa
- 1 can (15 oz) chickpeas, drained and rinsed
- 1 cup cherry tomatoes, halved
- 1 cucumber, diced
- 1/4 cup red onion, finely chopped
- Fresh parsley, chopped
- Feta cheese (optional)
- Lemon vinaigrette dressing

Instructions:

1. In a large bowl, combine cooked quinoa, chickpeas, cherry tomatoes, cucumber, and red onion.

2. Drizzle with lemon vinaigrette dressing and toss to combine.

3. Top with fresh parsley and feta cheese if desired.

Cooking Time: 15 minutes (if quinoa is pre-cooked)

2. Spinach and Mushroom Quesadilla

A quick and savory lunch option filled with leafy greens and earthy mushrooms.

Ingredients:

- Whole-grain tortilla
- 1 cup fresh spinach leaves
- 1/2 cup sliced mushrooms
- 1/4 cup shredded mozzarella cheese
- Olive oil for cooking
- Salt and pepper to taste

Instructions:

1. In a skillet, sauté the sliced mushrooms in olive oil until they're tender.

2. Add fresh spinach and cook until wilted.

3. Place the whole-grain tortilla in the skillet.

4. Add the sautéed mushrooms and spinach on one half of the tortilla.

5. Sprinkle with shredded mozzarella cheese and fold the tortilla in half.

6. Cook until the tortilla is crispy and the cheese is melted, flipping as needed.

Cooking Time: 10 minutes

3. Lentil and Vegetable Soup

A comforting and nutrient-rich soup that's perfect for a satisfying lunch.

Ingredients:

- 1 cup dried green or brown lentils, rinsed and drained
- 1 onion, chopped
- 2 carrots, diced
- 2 celery stalks, diced
- 2 cloves garlic, minced
- 6 cups vegetable broth
- 1 teaspoon dried thyme
- Salt and pepper to taste
- Fresh lemon juice (optional)

Instructions:

1. In a large pot, sauté the chopped onion, carrots, celery, and garlic until softened.

2. Add lentils, vegetable broth, dried thyme, salt, and pepper.

3. Bring to a boil, then reduce heat and simmer for about 30 minutes or until lentils are tender.

4. Add fresh lemon juice if desired before serving.

Cooking Time: 45 minutes

4. Grilled Chicken and Quinoa Bowl

This balanced bowl combines lean protein, whole grains, and colorful vegetables.

Ingredients:

- Grilled chicken breast
- 1 cup cooked quinoa
- Mixed greens
- Sliced bell peppers
- Cherry tomatoes
- Cucumber slices
- Balsamic vinaigrette dressing

Instructions:

1. Arrange mixed greens in a bowl.

2. Add cooked quinoa, grilled chicken breast, sliced bell peppers, cherry tomatoes, and cucumber slices.

3. Drizzle with balsamic vinaigrette dressing.

Cooking Time: 20 minutes (if quinoa is pre-cooked)

5. Sweet Potato and Chickpea Salad

This salad is a colorful mix of roasted sweet potatoes, chickpeas, and a zesty tahini dressing.

Ingredients:

- 2 sweet potatoes, peeled and cubed
- 1 can (15 oz) chickpeas, drained and rinsed
- Mixed greens
- Red onion, thinly sliced
- Tahini dressing
- Olive oil for roasting
- Salt, pepper, and paprika to taste

Instructions:

1. Toss sweet potato cubes with olive oil, salt, pepper, and paprika.

2. Roast in the oven at 400°F (200°C) for about 20-25 minutes until tender.

3. In a bowl, combine mixed greens, roasted sweet potatoes, chickpeas, and sliced red onion.

4. Drizzle with tahini dressing before serving.

Cooking Time: 30 minutes

6. Salmon and Asparagus Foil Packets

A simple and nutritious lunch option with omega-3-rich salmon and vibrant asparagus.

Ingredients:

- Salmon fillet
- Asparagus spears
- Lemon slices
- Fresh dill
- Olive oil
- Salt and pepper

Instructions:

1. Place a salmon fillet on a piece of foil.

2. Arrange asparagus spears around the salmon.

3. Drizzle with olive oil, season with salt and pepper, and add lemon slices and fresh dill on top.

4. Seal the foil packet and bake in the oven at 400°F (200°C) for about 15-20 minutes until salmon is cooked through.

Cooking Time: 20 minutes

7. Quinoa and Black Bean Stuffed Peppers

These stuffed peppers are filled with a protein-packed quinoa and black bean mixture.

Ingredients:

- Bell peppers (any color)
- 1 cup cooked quinoa
- 1 can (15 oz) black beans, drained and rinsed
- Corn kernels
- Salsa
- Shredded cheese (optional)

Instructions:

1. Cut the tops off the bell peppers and remove seeds and membranes.

2. In a bowl, combine cooked quinoa, black beans, corn kernels, and salsa.

3. Stuff the bell peppers with the quinoa mixture.

4. Sprinkle with shredded cheese if desired.

5. Bake in the oven at 375°F (190°C) for about 25-30 minutes until peppers are tender.

Cooking Time: 35 minutes (including baking time)

8. Veggie Stir-Fry with Tofu

A colorful stir-fry loaded with vegetables and protein-rich tofu.

Ingredients:

- Firm tofu, cubed
- Mixed stir-fry vegetables (bell peppers, broccoli, snap peas, carrots)
- Soy sauce or teriyaki sauce

- Garlic and ginger, minced

- Cooked brown rice or quinoa

Instructions:

1. In a skillet, stir-fry cubed tofu until browned.

2. Remove tofu from the skillet and set aside.

3. In the same skillet, stir-fry mixed vegetables with minced garlic and ginger.

4. Add tofu back to the skillet and drizzle with soy sauce or teriyaki sauce.

5. Serve over cooked brown rice or quinoa.

Cooking Time: 20 minutes (if rice or quinoa is pre-cooked)

9. Caprese Salad with Avocado

A refreshing and creamy take on the classic Caprese salad.

Ingredients:

- Ripe tomatoes, sliced

- Fresh mozzarella cheese, sliced

- Avocado, sliced

- Fresh basil leaves

- Balsamic glaze

- Olive oil

- Salt and pepper

Instructions:

1. Arrange sliced tomatoes, fresh mozzarella, and avocado on a plate.

2. Tuck fresh basil leaves between the slices.

3. Drizzle with balsamic glaze and olive oil.

4. Season with salt and pepper.

Cooking Time: 10 minutes

10. Tuna Salad Lettuce Wraps

A light and protein-packed lunch with a twist on traditional tuna salad.

Ingredients:

- Canned tuna, drained

- Greek yogurt

- Diced celery

- Diced red onion

- Dijon mustard

- Lettuce leaves (such as Bibb or Romaine)

- Sliced avocado

Instructions:

1. In a bowl, mix canned tuna with Greek yogurt, diced celery, diced red onion, and Dijon mustard.

2. Spoon the tuna salad into lettuce leaves.

3. Top with sliced avocado.

Cooking Time: 10 minutes

These lunch recipes are designed to provide you with a satisfying and nutritious midday meal while supporting your mental well-being. Adjust them to your preferences and dietary needs, and enjoy the flavors and benefits of these wholesome dishes.

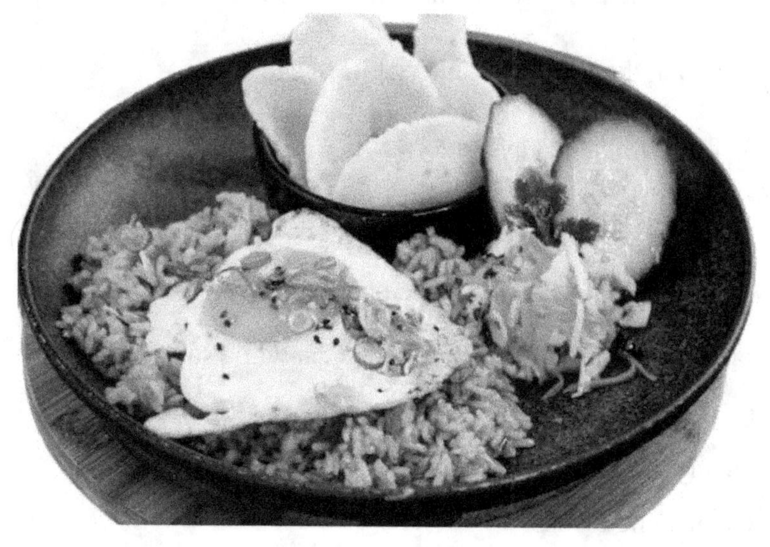

CHAPTER FOUR

Mental Health Diet Dinner Recipes

1. Baked Salmon with Lemon and Dill

Salmon is rich in omega-3 fatty acids, which are known to support mental health.

Ingredients:

- Salmon fillet
- Lemon slices
- Fresh dill
- Olive oil
- Salt and pepper

Instructions:

1. Place the salmon fillet on a baking sheet.

2. Drizzle with olive oil and season with salt and pepper.

3. Top with lemon slices and fresh dill.

4. Bake in the oven at 375°F (190°C) for 15-20 minutes or until the salmon flakes easily.

Cooking Time: 20 minutes

2. Roasted Vegetable and Chickpea Quinoa Bowl

This colorful bowl is packed with fiber, vitamins, and minerals.

Ingredients:

- Cooked quinoa
- Mixed roasted vegetables (bell peppers, zucchini, cherry tomatoes)
- Roasted chickpeas
- Fresh basil leaves
- Balsamic vinaigrette dressing

Instructions:

1. Arrange cooked quinoa, mixed roasted vegetables, and roasted chickpeas in a bowl.

2. Top with fresh basil leaves and drizzle with balsamic vinaigrette dressing.

Cooking Time: 30 minutes (if quinoa and roasted chickpeas are pre-cooked)

3. Turkey and Spinach Stuffed Bell Peppers

These stuffed peppers are a great source of lean protein and greens.

Ingredients:

- Bell peppers (any color)
- Ground turkey
- Fresh spinach leaves
- Quinoa or brown rice
- Tomato sauce
- Italian seasoning
- Shredded mozzarella cheese (optional)

Instructions:

1. Cut the tops off the bell peppers and remove seeds and membranes.

2. In a skillet, cook ground turkey until browned.

3. Add fresh spinach leaves and cook until wilted.

4. Mix in cooked quinoa or brown rice, tomato sauce, and Italian seasoning.

5. Stuff the bell peppers with the turkey and spinach mixture.

6. If desired, sprinkle with shredded mozzarella cheese.

7. Bake in the oven at 375°F (190°C) for about 25-30 minutes until peppers are tender.

Cooking Time: 45 minutes

4. Sautéed Shrimp with Garlic and Broccoli

Shrimp is a low-fat protein source, and broccoli is rich in vitamins and minerals.

Ingredients:

- Shrimp, peeled and deveined
- Broccoli florets
- Minced garlic
- Olive oil
- Lemon juice
- Salt and pepper

Instructions:

1. In a skillet, heat olive oil and sauté minced garlic until fragrant.

2. Add shrimp and cook until pink and opaque.

3. Add broccoli florets and cook until tender.

4. Drizzle with lemon juice and season with salt and pepper.

Cooking Time: 15 minutes

5. Veggie and Tofu Stir-Fry

A colorful stir-fry filled with vegetables and protein-rich tofu.

Ingredients:

- Firm tofu, cubed
- Mixed stir-fry vegetables (bell peppers, broccoli, snap peas, carrots)
- Soy sauce or teriyaki sauce
- Garlic and ginger, minced
- Cooked brown rice or quinoa

Instructions:

1. In a skillet, stir-fry cubed tofu until browned.

2. Remove tofu from the skillet and set aside.

3. In the same skillet, stir-fry mixed vegetables with minced garlic and ginger.

4. Add tofu back to the skillet and drizzle with soy sauce or teriyaki sauce.

5. Serve over cooked brown rice or quinoa.

Cooking Time: 20 minutes (if rice or quinoa is pre-cooked)

6. Baked Sweet Potato and Black Bean Tacos

Sweet potatoes provide complex carbs and black beans add protein and fiber.

Ingredients:

- Sweet potatoes, peeled and cubed
- Black beans, drained and rinsed
- Taco seasoning
- Whole-grain tortillas
- Sliced avocado
- Salsa
- Greek yogurt (as a sour cream alternative)

Instructions:

1. Toss sweet potato cubes with taco seasoning and roast in the oven at 400°F (200°C) for about 20-25 minutes until tender.

2. Warm whole-grain tortillas.

3. Fill tortillas with roasted sweet potatoes, black beans, sliced avocado, salsa, and a dollop of Greek yogurt.

Cooking Time: 30 minutes

7. Lemon Garlic Herb Chicken Breast

This simple chicken dish is bursting with flavor from lemon, garlic, and fresh herbs.

Ingredients:

- Chicken breast
- Lemon zest and juice
- Minced garlic
- Fresh herbs (rosemary, thyme, or parsley)
- Olive oil
- Salt and pepper

Instructions:

1. In a bowl, combine lemon zest, lemon juice, minced garlic, fresh herbs, olive oil, salt, and pepper.

2. Marinate chicken breast in the mixture for at least 30 minutes.

3. Grill or bake in the oven at 375°F (190°C) until the chicken is cooked through.

Cooking Time: 30 minutes

8. Lentil and Vegetable Curry

A comforting and flavorful curry filled with protein-packed lentils and a variety of vegetables.

Ingredients:

- Red lentils, rinsed and drained
- Mixed vegetables (bell peppers, cauliflower, carrots)
- Coconut milk
- Curry paste
- Fresh cilantro leaves
- Basmati rice

Instructions:

1. In a large pot, sauté mixed vegetables until they start to soften.

2. Add red lentils, coconut milk, and curry paste.

3. Simmer until lentils and vegetables are tender.

4. Serve over cooked basmati rice and garnish with fresh cilantro leaves.

Cooking Time: 45 minutes

9. Eggplant and Chickpea Stew

This hearty stew combines eggplant, chickpeas, and Mediterranean flavors.

Ingredients:

- Eggplant, cubed
- Chickpeas, drained and rinsed
- Diced tomatoes
- Onion, chopped
- Garlic cloves, minced

-   Olive oil

-   Cumin, paprika, and cinnamon

-   Fresh parsley leaves

Instructions:

1. In a large pot, sauté chopped onion and minced garlic in olive oil until translucent.

2. Add cubed eggplant and cook until it starts to soften.

3. Stir in diced tomatoes, chickpeas, and spices (cumin, paprika, and cinnamon).

4. Simmer until the eggplant is tender.

5. Garnish with fresh parsley leaves before serving.

Cooking Time: 40 minutes

10. Mushroom and Spinach Stuffed Chicken Breast

A delicious and elegant dish with protein-rich chicken and nutrient-packed spinach and mushrooms.

Ingredients:

- Chicken breast
- Fresh spinach leaves
- Sliced mushrooms
- Minced garlic
- Olive oil
- Feta cheese (optional)
- Salt and pepper

Instructions:

1. Butterfly the chicken breast by slicing it horizontally.

2. In a skillet, sauté sliced mushrooms and minced garlic in olive oil until mushrooms are browned.

3. Add fresh spinach leaves and cook until wilted.

4. Stuff the chicken breast with the mushroom and spinach mixture, and optionally, add feta cheese.

5. Secure with toothpicks or kitchen twine.

6. Season with salt and pepper.

7. Bake in the oven at 375°F (190°C) until the chicken is cooked through.

Cooking Time: 35 minutes

Mental Health Diet Snack Recipes

1. Mixed Berry Smoothie Bowl

A vibrant and antioxidant-rich snack that's perfect for boosting mood and concentration.

Ingredients:

- 1/2 cup mixed berries (strawberries, blueberries, raspberries)
- 1/2 ripe banana
- 1/2 cup Greek yogurt
- 1/4 cup almond milk
- Toppings: granola, sliced almonds, chia seeds, and honey

Instructions:

1. Blend mixed berries, banana, Greek yogurt, and almond milk until smooth.

2. Pour the smoothie into a bowl.

3. Top with granola, sliced almonds, chia seeds, and a drizzle of honey.

Preparation Time: 10 minutes

2. Guacamole with Veggie Sticks

Creamy avocado-based guacamole paired with colorful veggie sticks for a nutritious and mood-boosting snack.

Ingredients:

- 2 ripe avocados, mashed
- 1 tomato, diced
- 1/4 red onion, finely chopped
- 1 clove garlic, minced
- Lime juice
- Salt and pepper to taste
- Veggie sticks (carrots, celery, cucumber, bell peppers)

Instructions:

1. In a bowl, combine mashed avocados, diced tomato, chopped red onion, minced garlic, and a squeeze of lime juice.

2. Season with salt and pepper.

3. Serve with veggie sticks for dipping.

Preparation Time: 15 minutes

3. Greek Yogurt Parfait

A protein-packed parfait with the goodness of yogurt and fresh fruit to support your mental well-being.

Ingredients:

- Greek yogurt
- Mixed berries (strawberries, blueberries, raspberries)
- Granola
- Honey

Instructions:

1. In a glass or bowl, layer Greek yogurt, mixed berries, granola, and a drizzle of honey.

2. Repeat the layers as desired.

3. Serve immediately.

Preparation Time: 5 minutes

4. Almond Butter and Banana Toast

This snack combines healthy fats from almond butter with the natural sweetness of bananas on whole-grain toast.

Ingredients:

- Whole-grain bread
- Almond butter
- Sliced banana
- Honey (optional)

Instructions:

1. Toast whole-grain bread to your desired level of crispiness.

2. Spread almond butter on the toast.

3. Top with sliced banana.

4. Drizzle with honey if desired.

Preparation Time: 5 minutes

5. Cottage Cheese with Pineapple Chunks

A protein-rich and low-fat snack that includes the natural sweetness of pineapple.

Ingredients:

- Cottage cheese
- Pineapple chunks (fresh or canned)

Instructions:

1. In a bowl, scoop cottage cheese.

2. Top with pineapple chunks.

3. Enjoy as is or drizzle with a bit of pineapple juice.

Preparation Time: 2 minutes

6. Cucumber and Hummus Slices

A refreshing and crunchy snack with the hydrating benefits of cucumber and the protein-rich goodness of hummus.

Ingredients:

- Cucumber, sliced
- Hummus

Instructions:

1. Slice a cucumber into rounds or strips.

2. Serve with hummus for dipping.

Preparation Time: 5 minutes

7. Trail Mix with Nuts and Dried Fruits

A homemade trail mix combining nuts and dried fruits for a satisfying and nutritious snack.

Ingredients:

- Almonds
- Walnuts
- Cashews
- Dried cranberries

- Dried apricots, chopped
- Dark chocolate chips (optional)

Instructions:

1. Mix together almonds, walnuts, cashews, dried cranberries, dried apricots, and dark chocolate chips if desired.

2. Portion into snack-sized bags for easy grab-and-go.

Preparation Time: 5 minutes

8. Sliced Apples with Almond Butter

A simple yet satisfying snack that combines the crispness of apples with the creaminess of almond butter.

Ingredients:

- Apple, sliced
- Almond butter

Instructions:

1. Slice an apple into thin wedges.

2. Dip in almond butter before each bite.

Preparation Time: 5 minutes

9. Veggie Chips

Homemade baked veggie chips are a healthier alternative to traditional potato chips.

Ingredients:

- Sweet potatoes, beets, or zucchini, thinly sliced
- Olive oil
- Salt and pepper

Instructions:

1. Preheat the oven to 375°F (190°C).

2. Toss thinly sliced veggies with olive oil, salt, and pepper.

3. Spread them out on a baking sheet in a single layer.

4. Bake for about 20-30 minutes or until crispy, flipping halfway through.

Preparation Time: 35 minutes

10. Dark Chocolate-Covered Strawberries

A delightful and antioxidant-rich snack that satisfies your sweet tooth in a healthier way.

Ingredients:

- Strawberries
- Dark chocolate (70% cocoa or higher)

Instructions:

1. Melt dark chocolate in a microwave or on a stovetop using a double boiler.

2. Dip strawberries into the melted chocolate, covering them halfway.

3. Place on a parchment-lined tray and let them cool until the chocolate hardens.

Preparation Time: 15 minutes

These snack recipes are designed to be both delicious and beneficial for your mental health. Incorporate them into your daily routine to stay energized and focused throughout the day.

CONCLUSION

In conclusion, the significance of a mental health diet cannot be overstated. As our understanding of the intricate relationship between nutrition and mental well-being continues to evolve, it becomes increasingly evident that what we eat profoundly impacts not only our physical health but also our mental health.

A mental health diet is characterized by balance and mindfulness. It emphasizes whole, nutrient-dense foods such as fruits, vegetables, lean proteins, whole grains, and healthy fats. This diet provides the essential vitamins, minerals, antioxidants, and omega-3 fatty acids that are crucial for optimal brain function and emotional well-being.

The benefits of a mental health diet extend beyond just nourishing the brain. It plays a pivotal role in managing stress, anxiety, depression, and other mental health conditions.

Consuming foods rich in complex carbohydrates can boost serotonin production, promoting feelings of calm and contentment.

Omega-3 fatty acids found in fatty fish and flaxseeds have been linked to reduced symptoms of depression. Antioxidants in fruits and vegetables combat oxidative stress and inflammation, which are implicated in mood disorders.

Moreover, the gut-brain connection highlights the significance of a healthy digestive system in mental health. A diet rich in fiber and fermented foods supports a diverse gut microbiome, positively influencing mood regulation and reducing the risk of mental health issues.

While the benefits of a mental health diet are clear, it's essential to recognize that individual dietary needs can vary. Factors like genetics, allergies, and specific conditions may necessitate personalized approaches. Consulting with healthcare professionals and registered dietitians can help tailor dietary choices to individual circumstances.

Incorporating a mental health diet into one's lifestyle is not only about eating the right foods but also adopting mindful eating practices. Being present and attentive during meals, savoring the flavors and textures, and recognizing hunger and fullness cues are all integral components of mindful eating.

Ultimately, a mental health diet is a holistic approach to well-being, promoting not only a nourished body but also a resilient and balanced mind.

It empowers individuals to take an active role in their mental health, recognizing that what we put on our plates can contribute significantly to our overall happiness and emotional stability.

As we continue to explore the profound connection between nutrition and mental health, it is a reminder that making informed dietary choices is a powerful tool for nurturing our minds and fostering a brighter, more fulfilling future.

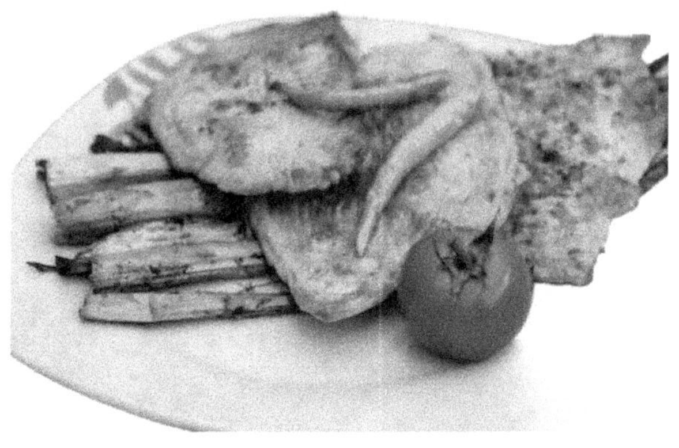

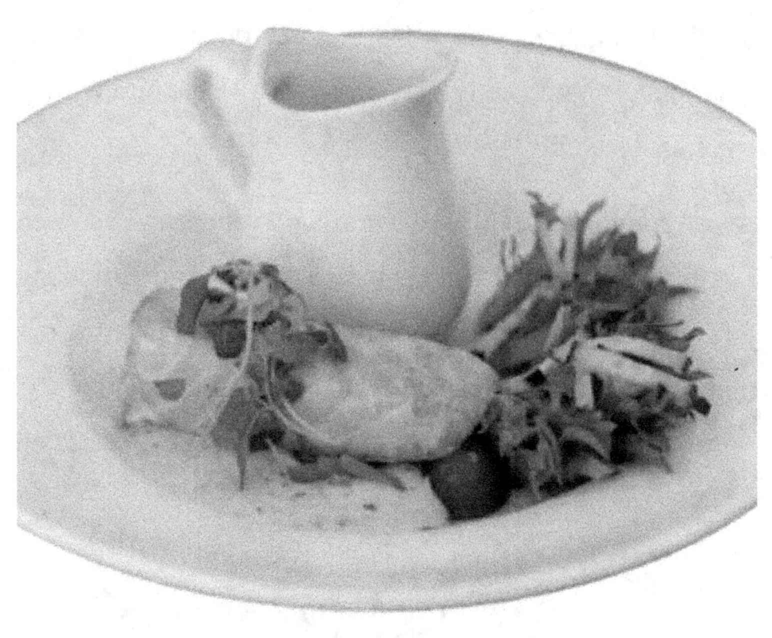